HOW TO LOSE WEIGHT WITHOUT EXERCISING

by Bobby V.

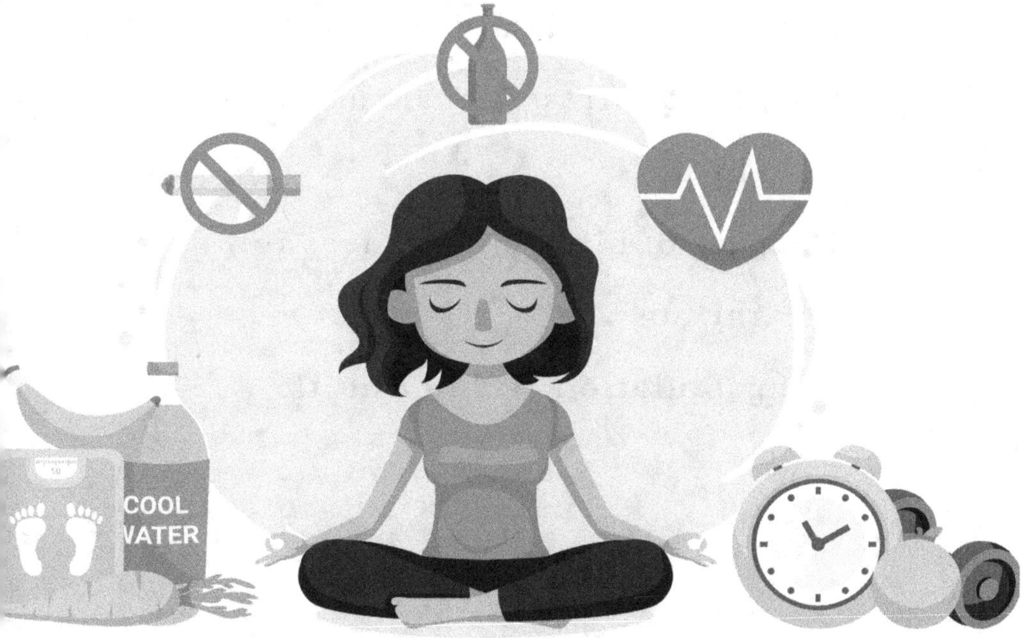

TABLE OF

CONTENTS

Click here for weight loss recipes!

INTRODUCTION

Losing weight is a common goal for many people, but not everyone wants to or is able to exercise. In this book, we will explore alternative methods for shedding unwanted pounds, without relying on physical activity.

We'll examine the science behind weight loss and look at strategies for making changes to your diet and lifestyle to support your goals.

Losing weight without exercise is possible but requires discipline and determination. The key to achieving weight loss without exercise is through managing caloric intake through a balanced diet and making lifestyle changes.

It's important to focus on consuming nutrient-dense foods and reducing empty calories from sources such as added sugars and saturated fats. Additionally, reducing sedentary behavior and increasing physical activity through daily movements can also contribute to weight loss.

While exercise is a crucial component of a healthy lifestyle and has numerous health benefits, weight loss can still be achieved through diet and lifestyle modifications alone.

CHAPTER 1: UNDERSTANDING WEIGHT LOSS

What is weight loss?

Weight loss refers to the process of reducing the total body mass, either by reducing body fat, muscle mass, or both. This can be achieved through a combination of diet, exercise, and other lifestyle changes.

The goal of weight loss is often to improve health, appearance, or both.

Factors that contribute to weight gain

There are several factors that can contribute to weight gain, including:

- Diet: Consuming more calories than your body burns, particularly from high-fat and high-sugar foods, can lead to weight gain.

- Lack of physical activity: Inactivity and sedentary behavior can contribute to weight gain, as the body burns fewer calories when it is not moving.

- Genetics: Genetics can play a role in weight gain by affecting factors such as metabolism and hunger levels.

- Medical conditions: Certain medical conditions, such as hypothyroidism, Cushing's syndrome, and polycystic ovary syndrome (PCOS), can cause weight gain.

- Medications: Some medications, such as

antidepressants and corticosteroids, can cause weight gain as a side effect.

- Stress: Chronic stress can lead to weight gain, as cortisol, the stress hormone, stimulates fat storage.

- Lack of sleep: Poor sleep habits can contribute to weight gain by affecting hormones that regulate hunger and metabolism.

The role of diet and lifestyle in weight loss

Diet and lifestyle play a crucial role in weight loss. Here's how:

- Diet: A calorie-controlled diet that focuses on whole, nutrient-dense foods can help you lose weight. It's important to limit the intake of high-fat and high-sugar foods and drinks, which can contribute to weight gain.

- Physical activity: Regular exercise can help you burn more calories, and thus, contribute to weight loss. Aim for at least 30 minutes of moderate physical activity, such as brisk walking, most days of the week.

- Hydration: Drinking adequate water can help boost metabolism and aid in weight loss.

- Sleep: Getting enough sleep (7-9 hours per night) can help regulate hormones that control hunger and metabolism, reducing the risk of weight gain.

- Stress management: Chronic stress can lead to weight gain, so it's important to manage stress through activities such as mindfulness, yoga, or exercise.

- Avoiding mindless eating: Mindless eating, such as snacking in front of the TV, can lead to overeating and weight gain. Instead, be mindful of portion sizes and limit distractions during meals.

Making lasting changes to your diet and lifestyle is crucial for successful weight loss and maintenance. It's important to work with a healthcare professional to develop a personalized plan that takes into account your individual needs and health status.

Understanding energy balance and metabolism

Energy balance refers to the balance between the energy (calories) you consume through food and drinks, and the energy you use through physical activity and metabolism.

If you consume more calories than your body uses, you will gain weight, and if you consume fewer calories than your body uses, you will lose weight.

Metabolism refers to the processes by which your body converts food into energy and uses that energy for various functions, such as breathing, digestion, and physical activity. Your metabolism is influenced by several factors, including genetics, age, sex, muscle mass, and physical activity levels.

A slower metabolism means that your body burns fewer calories at rest, making it easier to gain weight. Conversely, a faster metabolism means that your body burns more calories at rest, making it easier to maintain a healthy weight.

Energy balance and metabolism play a critical role in weight management. To achieve and
maintain a healthy weight, it's important to maintain number of calories for your individual needs and being physically active.

CHAPTER 2: NUTRITION FOR WEIGHT LOSS

Nutrition plays a crucial role in weight loss. To lose weight, it's important to create a calorie deficit, which means consuming fewer calories than the body burns. A balanced diet that includes a variety of nutrient-dense foods is essential for weight loss.

Here are some key nutrients and foods that can help with weight loss:

1. Protein: High-protein foods take longer to digest, keeping you full for longer. Examples include chicken, fish, eggs, and legumes.

2. Fiber: Foods high in fiber, such as fruits, vegetables, and whole grains, slow down digestion and help you feel full.

3. Healthy fats: Foods such as avocados, nuts, and olive oil can help reduce hunger and increase fullness.

4. Water: Drinking water before meals can help reduce calorie intake and increase feelings of fullness.

5. Low-calorie, nutrient-dense foods: Foods such as leafy greens, berries, and carrots are low in calories but high in nutrients and can help you feel full.

In addition, it's important to avoid highly processed foods, sugary drinks, and excessive amounts of added sugars, as these can lead to weight gain and other health problems.

Remember, sustainable weight loss requires a balanced, calorie-controlled diet combined with physical activity. Consult a registered dietitian for personalized advice.

Importance of a balanced diet

A balanced diet is important for overall health and wellness, as well as for weight management.
A balanced diet includes a variety of nutrient-dense foods from all food groups, including:

1. Fruits and vegetables: These provide essential vitamins, minerals, and fiber.

2. Whole grains: Whole grains are a good source of fiber, which can help regulate digestion and control blood sugar levels.

3. Lean protein: Protein is essential for building and repairing muscle, and also helps regulate hunger and fullness.

4. Healthy fats: Healthy fats such as those found in nuts, seeds, and oily fish provide energy and help absorb certain vitamins.

5. Dairy or dairy alternatives: These provide calcium and other important nutrients for bone health.

By consuming a variety of nutrient-dense foods, you can ensure that your body is getting all the nutrients it needs to function optimally. This can help reduce the risk of chronic diseases and support overall health.

Additionally, a balanced diet can help maintain a healthy weight, reduce feelings of hunger and increase feelings of fullness.

Understanding macronutrients and micronutrients

Macronutrients and micronutrients are essential components of a balanced diet. Macronutrients are the nutrients that the body requires in large quantities and include:

Carbohydrates: These provide the body with energy and are found in foods such as grains, fruits, and vegetables.

Proteins: These are essential for building and repairing tissues and can be found in foods such as meat, poultry, fish, eggs, dairy, and legumes.

Fats: These are a source of energy and help absorb certain vitamins. Good sources of healthy fats include nuts, seeds, and oily fish.

Micronutrients, on the other hand, are vitamins and minerals that the body needs in smaller quantities. Examples include:

Vitamins: Such as vitamins A, C, D, and E, which are important for overall health, growth, and development.

Minerals: Such as iron, calcium, and magnesium, which are essential for maintaining strong bones, supporting muscle function, and regulating bodily processes.

Both macronutrients and micronutrients are important for optimal health and should be included in a balanced diet. The exact balance of macronutrients required by an individual will depend on their age, gender, and activity level. A registered dietitian can help develop a personalized eating plan that meets an individual's specific needs.

Limiting calorie-dense, nutritionally-poor foods

Limiting calorie-dense, nutritionally-poor foods is an important part of a balanced diet for weight management and overall health. Such foods are often high in added sugars, unhealthy fats, and refined carbohydrates and are low in essential nutrients. Examples include:

Junk food: Such as chips, candy, and processed snacks, which are high in calories and low in nutrients.

Sugary drinks: Such as soda, sports drinks, and fruit juice, which are high in added sugars and calories.

Highly processed foods: Such as white bread, crackers, and frozen dinners, which are low in fiber and nutrients.

Consuming large amounts of these foods can lead to

weight gain, as they provide a lot of calories but little nutritional value. Additionally, they can increase the risk of chronic diseases such as type 2 diabetes and heart disease.

To limit calorie-dense, nutritionally-poor foods, try to focus on eating a diet rich in whole, nutrient-dense foods. Incorporate plenty of fruits, vegetables, whole grains, lean protein, and healthy fats into your meals and snacks. Additionally, it may be helpful to limit portion sizes and avoid overeating, as well as to limit added sugars and unhealthy fats.

Incorporating nutrient-dense, low calorie foods

Incorporating nutrient-dense, low calorie foods into your diet can help support weight loss and overall health. Nutrient-dense foods are those that provide a high amount of nutrients for a low number of calories. Examples include:

Fruits and vegetables: These are low in calories but high in fiber, vitamins, and minerals. Try to include a variety of colors in your diet for maximum nutrient diversity.

Whole grains: Such as brown rice, quinoa, and whole wheat bread, are a good source of fiber and other nutrients.

Lean protein: Such as chicken, fish, tofu, and legumes, can help regulate hunger and fullness and provide important nutrients for muscle building and repair.

Nuts and seeds: These are a good source of healthy fats, protein, and fiber.

Low-fat dairy: Such as milk, yogurt, and cheese, provide calcium and other important nutrients for bone health.

Incorporating these foods into your diet can help you feel full and satisfied while reducing your overall calorie intake. To make it easier, try incorporating these foods into your meals and snacks, and replacing less nutritious options with healthier alternatives. A registered dietitian can help develop a personalized eating plan that incorporates nutrient-dense, low calorie foods and supports your weight loss goals.

Hydration and its impact on weight loss

Hydration is important for overall health and can have a significant impact on weight loss. Drinking enough water can help regulate digestion, control hunger and fullness, and increase feelings of satiety. In addition, drinking water can also help flush out excess sodium and toxins from the body, which can reduce bloating and help with weight loss.

However, it's important to be mindful of what you're drinking, as sugary drinks and drinks high in calories can contribute to weight gain. Water is the best option for hydration, and you can also consider unsweetened tea, sparkling water, and 100% fruit juice in moderation.

A general guideline for hydration is to aim for 8-8 ounces of water per day. However, individual needs may vary based on factors such as age, gender, physical activity level, and climate. To ensure you're getting enough hydration, you can check the color of your urine. Light yellow or clear urine is a sign of adequate hydration, while darker yellow urine may indicate the need to drink more fluids.

CHAPTER 3: MINDFUL EATING AND HUNGER MANAGEMENT

Mindful eating is a concept that involves paying attention to one's physical and emotional sensations while eating, in order to develop a more conscious and healthy relationship with food. It helps in recognizing true hunger and fullness signals, reducing mindless snacking and overeating, and ultimately promoting physical and mental well-being.

Hunger management involves understanding the underlying factors that drive hunger, such as physiological need, emotions, or habits. By identifying these drivers, one can develop strategies to better manage their hunger, such as eating regularly scheduled meals, finding alternative ways to manage emotions, or practicing mindfulness.

Overall, mindful eating and hunger management go hand in hand in promoting a healthier relationship with food and reducing the risk of overeating and weight gain.

Understanding your relationship with food

Understanding one's relationship with food is a critical component of mindful eating and hunger management. It involves recognizing the emotional, psychological, and social factors that influence food choices and habits. This may include exploring past experiences, family dynamics, cultural influences, and current emotional states that may impact eating habits.

It also involves recognizing the role of food in one's life and its impact on physical, mental, and emotional well-being. This can help in developing a healthier relationship with food and reducing disordered eating patterns.

Ultimately, understanding your relationship with food can lead to increased self-awareness and provide insight into why you eat the way you do. With this understanding, you can make more mindful and intentional food choices that better align with your physical and emotional needs.

Identifying and overcoming emotional eating

Emotional eating refers to using food as a way to cope with emotions, such as stress, boredom, or anxiety, rather than to satisfy physical hunger. It can lead to overeating and weight gain and have negative effects on physical and emotional health.

To identify emotional eating, it's important to become aware of triggers and patterns. Keeping a food diary that tracks what you eat, how much you eat, and how you're feeling at the time can be helpful in identifying patterns of emotional eating.

To overcome emotional eating, it's important to develop alternative coping strategies. Some strategies include:

Practicing mindfulness and self-awareness: Paying

attention to physical hunger and fullness cues, and understanding the emotions and triggers that lead to emotional eating.

Finding alternative coping mechanisms: Engaging in physical activity, deep breathing, meditation, or talking to a trusted friend or therapist to manage stress and negative emotions.

Challenging negative thought patterns: Identifying and reframing negative thoughts and beliefs about food and body image that contribute to emotional eating.

Fostering a healthy relationship with food: Learning to eat mindfully and intuitively, and avoiding food restriction and deprivation.

Remember that overcoming emotional eating is a journey, and it's important to be kind and compassionate with yourself. Seeking support from a therapist or a support group can also be helpful in overcoming emotional eating and developing a healthier relationship with food.

Strategies for mindful eating and portion control

- Mindful eating and portion control are important strategies for promoting a healthy relationship with food and preventing overeating. Here are some practical tips for incorporating these principles into your daily life:

- Practice mindfulness: Pay attention to the experience of eating, including the taste, texture, and smell of food, and how it makes you feel physically and emotionally.

- Eat slowly and savor each bite: Put down your utensils between bites and chew thoroughly. This can help you feel full faster and enjoy your food more.

- Listen to your body's hunger and fullness signals: Eat when you're hungry and stop when you're satisfied, rather than eating until you're full.

- Avoid distractions while eating: Turn off the TV and put away your phone, and focus on the experience of eating.

- Use smaller plates and bowls: Research has shown that using smaller dishes can help you eat less without feeling deprived.

- Plan meals and snacks in advance: Having a plan can help you make healthier food choices and prevent overeating.

- Serve yourself smaller portions: Use measuring cups or a kitchen scale to ensure that you're eating appropriate portions.

- Avoid skipping meals: Skipping meals can lead to overeating later in the day, so aim to eat three meals and two snacks daily.

By incorporating these strategies into your daily life, you can develop a healthier relationship with food and prevent overeating, ultimately leading to better physical and emotional well-being.

Planning ahead to avoid impulsive eating decisions

Impulsive eating decisions often result from a lack of planning and preparation, leading to unhealthy food choices or overeating. To avoid this, it's important to plan ahead and have healthy options readily available. Here are some tips to help:

- Plan your meals and snacks: Make a grocery list and stick to it. Include healthy options like fruits, vegetables, whole grains, and lean proteins.

- Pack your own meals and snacks: Bring a healthy lunch and snacks to work or school, rather than relying on fast food or vending machines.

- Keep healthy snacks on hand: Stock your pantry and refrigerator with healthy snack options, like cut-up vegetables, fruit, or yogurt.

- Cook in bulk: Cook larger portions of healthy meals and freeze the leftovers for future meals.

- Avoid shopping when you're hungry: Shop for groceries after you've had a meal to avoid impulse buys.

- Stay hydrated: Drink plenty of water, especially before meals, to avoid overeating.

By planning ahead and having healthy options readily available, you can make more informed and mindful food choices and prevent impulsive eating decisions. This, in turn, can help in developing a healthier relationship with food and reducing the risk of overeating and weight gain.

CHAPTER 4: SLEEP AND WEIGHT LOSS

Sleep and weight loss are interconnected. Lack of sleep can lead to weight gain by affecting hormones that regulate hunger and metabolism, causing cravings for high-calorie foods, and reducing physical activity levels.

On the other hand, getting adequate and quality sleep can help with weight loss by improving energy levels, reducing stress, and allowing for better self-control and decision-making. It is recommended to get 7-9 hours of sleep per night and establish a consistent sleep schedule to support weight loss goals.

Understanding the link between sleep and weight loss

The link between sleep and weight loss is complex and multifaceted. Poor sleep can disrupt the hormones responsible for regulating hunger (ghrelin) and fullness (leptin), leading to increased appetite and cravings for high-calorie, sugary foods. Additionally, lack of sleep can reduce energy levels and motivation for physical activity, leading to decreased calorie burn.

On the other hand, adequate and quality sleep can help support weight loss by reducing stress and promoting better decision-making and self-control, which can result in healthier food choices and more physical activity. It can also help regulate hormones and metabolism, which can contribute to weight management.

It is important to note that while sleep is a crucial factor in weight management, it should not be the only focus. A balanced diet, regular physical activity, and healthy lifestyle habits also play a significant role in promoting weight loss.

Tips for improving your sleep quality and duration

Here are some tips to improve your sleep quality and duration:

- Establish a consistent sleep schedule: Try to go to bed and wake up at the same time every day, even on weekends.

- Create a sleep-conducive environment: Keep your bedroom cool, dark, and quiet, and invest in a comfortable mattress and pillows.

- Limit screen time before bed: The blue light from electronic devices can interfere with sleep, so avoid using them for at least an hour before bedtime.

- Avoid caffeine and alcohol before bedtime: Both can interfere with sleep quality, so limit consumption or avoid them in the hours leading up to bedtime.

- Exercise regularly: Regular physical activity can improve sleep quality and help you fall asleep faster, but be sure to finish exercising a few hours before bedtime.

- Practice relaxation techniques: Try techniques like deep breathing, meditation, or yoga to help calm your mind and prepare for sleep.

- Avoid naps during the day: Napping can interfere with nighttime sleep, so try to avoid it or limit it to no more than 20-30 minutes in the early afternoon.

By incorporating these tips into your daily routine, you can improve your sleep quality and duration, which can support your weight loss goals.

The impact of sleep deprivation on weight gain

Sleep deprivation can have a significant impact on weight gain. When you don't get enough sleep, it can disrupt the hormones that regulate hunger and metabolism, causing an increase in hunger and cravings for high-calorie, sugary foods. This can lead to overeating and weight gain.

Additionally, lack of sleep can reduce energy levels, making it more difficult to engage in physical activity and burning fewer calories. Furthermore, sleep deprivation can increase levels of the hormone cortisol, which is associated with stress and has been linked to abdominal fat accumulation.

Finally, poor sleep can also affect cognitive function, making it more difficult to make healthy choices and exercise self-control, further contributing to weight gain.

Therefore, it is important to prioritize sleep and aim for 7-9 hours of quality sleep each night to support weight loss and overall health.

CHAPTER 5: STRESS MANAGEMENT AND WEIGHT LOSS

Stress and weight loss are often interconnected. Stressful events or chronic stress can lead to overeating or unhealthy food choices, which can contribute to weight gain. On the other hand, excess weight can also contribute to stress and low self-esteem.

To manage stress and support weight loss, it's important to engage in regular physical activity, eat a balanced diet, get enough sleep, and practice stress-management techniques such as mindfulness, deep breathing, or yoga. Additionally, seeking support from friends and family or a mental health professional can also be beneficial.

It's important to remember that weight loss and stress management are ongoing processes, and progress may be slow. It's essential to be patient and persistent, and to make lifestyle changes that are sustainable in the long-term.

Understanding the impact of stress on weight

Stress can impact weight in several ways. Chronic stress can lead to an increase in cortisol, a hormone that can cause an increase in appetite, particularly for high-fat, high-sugar foods. This can result in overeating and weight gain. Stress can also disrupt sleep patterns, which can lead to fatigue and decreased physical activity, further contributing to weight gain.

In addition, stress can cause a decrease in physical activity as people may lack the energy or motivation to exercise. This, in combination with unhealthy eating habits, can lead to weight gain.

On the other hand, stress can also cause weight loss as a result of stress-related behaviors such as skipping meals, binge eating, or engaging in excessive physical activity. It's important to manage stress in a healthy way to avoid these negative impacts on weight.

Strategies for managing stress and reducing cortisol levels

There are several effective strategies for managing stress and reducing cortisol levels:

Exercise: Regular physical activity, such as running, hiking, yoga or strength training, can help manage stress and lower cortisol levels.

Relaxation techniques: Practicing mindfulness, deep breathing, or meditation can help calm the mind and reduce stress.

Sleep: Getting adequate sleep is important for overall health, including reducing stress levels and regulating cortisol levels. Aim for 7-9 hours of sleep per night.

Healthy eating: Consuming a balanced diet that includes plenty of fruits, vegetables, whole grains, and lean protein can support stress management and help regulate cortisol levels.

Social support: Having a supportive network of friends, family, or a mental health professional can help individuals manage stress and cope with difficult situations.

Time management: Prioritizing and organizing daily tasks can help reduce stress levels and promote a sense of control.

Reduce caffeine and alcohol intake: Caffeine and alcohol can disrupt cortisol levels and contribute to feelings of stress and anxiety. Limiting or eliminating these substances can help reduce cortisol levels and manage stress.

It's important to find what works best for each individual and to make stress management a priority in daily life.

Mind-body practices for stress reduction, such as meditation and yoga

Yes, mind-body practices such as meditation and yoga can be effective for reducing stress.

Meditation: Meditation is a practice that involves focusing the mind on the present moment, often through deep breathing and mindfulness. Research has shown that meditation can help reduce stress and anxiety, lower cortisol levels, and improve overall well-being.

Yoga: Yoga combines physical postures, breathing exercises, and meditation to promote relaxation and stress relief. Practicing yoga can help reduce cortisol levels, lower stress, and improve physical and mental well-being.

Both meditation and yoga are easily accessible, low-cost and can be practiced anywhere, making them accessible stress-management tools for people of all ages and abilities. It's important to find a practice that feels comfortable and enjoyable, as consistency and enjoyment are key to experiencing the full benefits of these mind-body practices.

CHAPTER 6: LIFESTYLE CHANGES FOR WEIGHT LOSS

Lifestyle changes are essential for long-term weight loss success. Here are some tips:

Eating a balanced diet: Focus on consuming a variety of nutrient-dense foods, such as fruits, vegetables, lean protein, and whole grains.

Monitoring calorie intake: Keep track of the number of calories you consume daily to ensure you are not overloading your body with more energy than it needs.

Incorporating physical activity into your daily routine, without formal exercise

There are many ways to incorporate physical activity into your daily routine without doing formal exercise. Some examples include:

- Take the stairs instead of the elevator or escalator.

- Walk or cycle to work or run errands instead of driving.

- Stand up and stretch every hour while working at your desk.

- Take frequent breaks during the day to walk around the office or outside.

- Do household chores like cleaning and gardening.

- Play with your children or pets, go for a walk with friends, or join a recreational sports team.

- Try an active hobby like dancing, hiking, or rock climbing.

Remember, even small amounts of physical activity can add up over the course of a day and have a positive impact on your health.

Staying hydrated: Drinking plenty of water helps regulate hunger and flush out toxins from the body.

Getting enough sleep: Aim for 7-9 hours of sleep per night. Lack of sleep can lead to hormonal imbalances that increase appetite and decrease metabolism.

Managing stress: Chronic stress can lead to overeating and weight gain, so finding healthy ways to manage stress is important.

Avoiding fad diets and quick fixes: Sustainable weight loss is achieved through gradual changes to your lifestyle and habits, not through extreme diets or quick fixes.

Remember, making lifestyle changes is a journey and it may take time to see results. Be patient and consistent, and focus on progress rather than perfection.

Making sustainable changes to your diet and lifestyle is crucial for long-term weight loss success

Here are some tips for making sustainable changes:

Start small: Make gradual changes to your diet and exercise routine to make it easier to stick to.

Find what works for you: Experiment with different eating and exercise styles to find what works best for you and your lifestyle.

Make it a habit: Incorporating healthy habits into your daily routine makes it easier to stick to in the long term.

Plan ahead: Plan your meals and snacks in advance to avoid reaching for unhealthy options when you're in a rush or hungry.

Get support: Surround yourself with people who support your goals and hold you accountable. Consider joining a support group or working with a dietitian or personal trainer.

Stay positive: Focusing on the positive changes you are making, rather than the number on the scale, can help keep you motivated.

Celebrate your successes: Celebrate your milestones and accomplishments along the way, no matter how small they may be.

Remember, weight loss is a journey and it may take time to see results. Be patient, persistent, and focus on making healthy lifestyle changes that you can maintain for life.

Staying motivated and accountable to your weight loss goals

Staying motivated and accountable to your weight loss goals can be challenging, but it's essential for success. Here are some tips:

Set realistic goals: Start with small, achievable goals and work your way up. This will help you build momentum and stay motivated.

Keep track of your progress: Keep a food diary or log your weight regularly to see your progress and stay accountable.

Find a workout buddy: Exercise is more fun with a friend, and having someone to hold you accountable can be a great motivator.

Reward yourself: Treat yourself to something special when you reach a milestone or achieve a goal, such as a massage, a new outfit, or a night out with friends.

Stay positive: Focus on the progress you're making and the healthy habits you're developing, rather than the setbacks.

Stay flexible: Be willing to adjust your goals and plans if necessary, but don't give up on your overall vision of a healthier, happier you.

Get support: Surround yourself with people who

support your goals and hold you accountable. Consider joining a support group or working with a dietitian or personal trainer.

YOU DID IT!
THIS IS THE FIRST MAJOR STEP

Weight loss without exercising is a achievable goal that can be achieved through a combination of diet and lifestyle changes. By reducing caloric intake, focusing on nutrient-dense foods, and increasing physical activity through daily movements, weight loss can be successfully attained.

While regular exercise is important for overall health and weight maintenance, weight loss can still be achieved without it. It is essential to consult a healthcare professional to create a personalized approach to weight loss that is safe and effective.

With the right mindset, diet and lifestyle changes, anyone can reach their weight loss goals without relying solely on exercise.

Remember to celebrate your successes along the way and be kind to yourself when setbacks occur. Stay focused and motivated, and you'll reach your goals in no time.

You are now officially on your personal health and weight loss journey!

If you're interested in healthy weight loss friendly meals, check out this YouTube channel on plant-based recipes!

Click here for weight loss recipes!